Table of Contents

Lunch

Greek Salad

Mediterranean Quinoa Salad

Creamy White Bean Soup

Pasta Fagioli Soup

Barley Salad

Dinner

Mediterranean Stew, Slow-Cooker Style

Mediterranean Flounder

Shrimp Penne

Greek Chicken Pasta

Red Pepper and Rosemary Chicken, Slow Cooker Style

Dessert

Orange and Olive Oil Cake

Mediterranean Diet

Easy Recipes for A Healthy Diet And Permanent Weight Loss By Cooking Delicious Meals

Greek Yogurt with Honey, Walnuts, and Figs

Mango-Watermelon Mint Slushy

Conclusion

Introduction

The typical western diet is packed full of sugar, salt, and fat and the combination of those three is explosively unhealthy. Obesity is on the rise if you will forgive the pun, so are instances of heart disease, cognitive decline and many other medical conditions and health risks, all associated with our diets.

That is why so many people are turning to The Mediterranean Diet. This is more than just a diet; this is a way of life that is firmly based in traditional Mediterranean foods and drinks. Unlike many other so-called diets, the Mediterranean diet allows you to live your life freely, without restriction. You can join your friends and family for a meal or go to a restaurant without having to worry too much about what you are eating.

The Mediterranean diet brings together the culture and traditions of countries like Greece, Spain, Italy, and France, providing you with a wide variety of foods to choose from. While Mediterranean cuisine varies from country to country and even region to region within a country, it is mostly based on fruit, vegetables, nuts, cereal grains, fish and olive oil, with little meat being consumed.

Mediterranean cuisine varies by region and has a range of definitions, but is largely based on vegetables, fruits, nuts, beans, cereal grains, olive oil, and fish. And let's not forget a good drop of red wine to wash it all down with.

If you are ready to try something that has been around for years, a diet that has been proven time and time again to be the healthiest in the world, then you have come to the right place. You are about to start a new journey; a journey where you train your body to forget about processed foods full of fat and sugar and learn to enjoy foods that are full of essential nutrients, natural foods that take us back to how we used to live.

Thank you for choosing to read my book. I hope that I am able to provide you with the information you need, along with a few delicious recipes that tempt you into changing your way of life to a Mediterranean one.

Chapter 1: What is the Mediterranean Diet?

When we think of a Mediterranean diet, many of us immediately think of pasta and pizza in Italy or pita and hummus in Greece. Sadly, like the rack of lamb, lasagna, falafel and gyros that we automatically associate with the Mediterranean, none of these foods are healthy and none of them feature in the true Mediterranean diet.

The reality is the Mediterranean diet consists of whole foods – fruits, vegetables, olive oil, seafood, whole grains and other healthy foods that can help to fight against chronic diseases like diabetes and heart disease, some cancers and even cognitive decline. This is truly a diet worth going for, although making the change from meaty lasagnas and pepperoni pizza to salmon and avocado might take some doing, it is truly worth the effort.

Following the end of the Second World War, an American scientist by the name of Ancel Keys studied the health and the diets of about 13,000 middle-aged males from Greece, the US, Italy, Japan, Finland, the Netherlands and Yugoslavia. What he found was that the American men who ate a hearty diet had much higher rates of heart diseases than those from the countries where war deprivation had restricted their diets. The poorest men in the study were those who lived on the Greek island of Crete and they had the best rates of cardiovascular health, due to two things – hard physical labor and a unique food pyramid.

The Mediterranean Pyramid is based on the traditional diets of Greece, Crete, and Italy from the 1960's, at a time when their populations showed the lowest rates of heart disease and other chronic diseases and the highest life expectancy, despite a lack of medical services. Aside from the food that they eat, a diet of fresh food and homegrown food, the other important elements to their diet are exercise on a daily basis, eating their meals with others and a truly deep appreciation for the delicious and healthy foods that they eat.

The General Principles of the Mediterranean Diet

The Mediterranean diet is not about superfoods that are a "quick fix". Nor is it a strict list of the foods you should avoid, like so many other diets out there today. Instead, the Mediterranean diet is a proper formula for eating healthily on a daily basis for the long-term, not just the two weeks it takes to shift the pounds that you want to drop. The following are the general principles of the Mediterranean diet, a guide for all of you who want to give this a go:

- Eat more vegetables, beans, peas, whole grain cereals, and fruits

- Limit how much red meat you eat – instead, eat poultry or fish

- Where you can, use rapeseed or olive oil – monounsaturated fats – rather that animal fats like lard and butter

- Restrict how much highly processed food you eat, such as ready meals and fast foods that may be loaded with saturated fat, sugar, and salt.

- Limit your intake of dairy products and go for low-fat versions

- Never add extra salt to your meals at the table – there is already enough in the food

- If you want a snack, go for unsalted nuts, dried fruit and fresh fruit instead of crisps, cakes, and biscuits

- Drink no more than 2 small glasses of red wine per day, preferably with your meals

- Forget sugary sodas; when you want a non-alcoholic drink, go for water. Small amounts of tea and coffee are ok but not loaded with milk, cream, and sugar.

Chapter 2: The Benefits of the Mediterranean Diet

So, what are the benefits of the Mediterranean diet and how do they affect you?

1. Low in Sugar and Processed Foods

The Mediterranean diet consists of ingredients that are as close to nature as you can possibly get. These include legumes, olive oil, vegetables, fruits, unrefined cereals and small amounts of animal product. All of these foods should be locally grown and organic. In contrast to the typical western diet, this one is low in sugar and contains almost no artificial ingredients or GMOs, no preservatives, and no flavor enhancers. If you have a sweet tooth, choose fruit and honey. Wild caught fish and a low consumption of yogurts and cheeses made from goat, cow or sheep milk are a good way to get your daily dose of good fats and cholesterol and fish like sardines and anchovies are a big part of the Mediterranean diet. Low meat consumption and light meals are the order of the day, with fish the main part of many meals as this improves your intake of omega 3, and improves cholesterol and the health of your heart.

2. Lose Weight the Healthy Way

If you want to lose weight without a restriction in food or feeling hungry all the time, and if you want to maintain that weight once you reach it, the Mediterranean is a good plan. It is a sustainable diet, one that you can eat for the rest of your life without feeling like you are missing out on something. The Mediterranean diet is the most successful in the world for helping to reduce your intake of fat and managing weight with nutrient-dense food choices.

This is a flexible diet. You can choose to eat low carb, low protein or somewhere in the middle because the diet concentrates on eating healthy fats and keeping carbohydrate levels down while increasing your intake of healthy and high-quality proteins. If you wanted to eat protein rather than grains or legumes you can lose weight in a healthy way, with no deprivation, eating high-quality dairy and fish. On the other hand, vegetarians can benefit from the Mediterranean diet as well, with a wide range of fruits, vegetables, legumes, and grains to choose from.

3. It Improves Your Heart Health

Research has shown that, when people stick to the Mediterranean diet, eating plenty of omega-3 and monounsaturated fats, the risk of heart disease is dramatically reduced. Take olive oil, for example. It contains alpha-linoleic acid (ALA) and this has been shown, time and time again, to cut the risk of death from heart disease by 30% and the rates of death from sudden heart attack by 45%. Research also shows that blood pressure is measurably lower in people who consume olive oil as opposed to sunflower oil. Another reason that olive oil is good for lowering blood pressure is that it makes nitric oxide far more bioavailable and this means that your arteries are kept dilated and clearer. It also fights against oxidation, an effect that promotes disease.

4. It Can Help to Fight Cancer

The European Journal of Cancer Prevention says that "*The biological mechanisms for cancer prevention associated with the Mediterranean diet have been related to the favorable effect of a balanced ratio of omega-6 and omega-3 essential fatty acids and high amounts of fiber, antioxidants and polyphenols found in fruit, vegetables, olive oil and wine.*"

The building blocks of the Mediterranean diet are vegetables and fruits and it is plant foods like these that fight cancer in just about every way possible – by providing antioxidants, by stopping cells from mutating, by protecting our DNA from being damaged and by reducing inflammation and slowing down the growth of tumors.

There are also a lot of studies pointing to olive oil being a possible natural cure for cancer, in particular, colon and bowel cancer. It could be that the oil stops cancer cells from forming because it lowers inflammation and cuts down on stress caused by oxidation.

5. It Can Help to Treat or Prevent Diabetes

There is evidence to suggest that the Mediterranean diet can help to fight off chronic diseases that are related to inflammation, such as Metabolic Syndrome and Type 2 diabetes. One main reason that this diet is so beneficial is that it reduces insulin, the hormone that controls our glucose levels and is what makes us put on weight and keep it on, no matter how many diets we go on.

By regulating glucose levels using natural whole foods, the body is able to use fat reserves for energy more efficiently and, as such, a diet low in sugar with good fats and fresh whole foods can be seen as a natural cure for diabetes. The AHA (American Heart

Association) says that, while the Mediterranean diet is higher in fat than a standard western diet, it is lower in saturated fats. It is normally a rough ratio of 20-30% high-quality protein, 30-40% healthy fat and 40% complex carbohydrates. This is the ideal balance for keeping hunger under control and is a good way for the body to regular insulin production or stay in hormonal homeostasis. A result of this is that moods are higher and physical activity levels are increased along with energy.

6. It Can Help to Prevent Cognitive Diseases

The Mediterranean diet may also be seen as a natural form of treatment for Alzheimer's, Parkinson's, and some forms of dementia. These kinds of cognitive disorders occur when your brain does no receive enough dopamine. This is a chemical that is vital for proper movement in the body, thought processing and mood regulation.

Healthy fats and anti-inflammatory vegetables and fruits have been shown to fight cognitive decline that is related to age. They help to fight against the harmful effects of free radicals, exposure to toxins, food allergies and the inflammation caused by a poor diet, all of which play a part in brain function impairment and adhering to the Mediterranean diet has long been shown to have a link to reducing the chances of Alzheimer's disease.

7. It Can Help to Prolong Life Expectancy

Diets that are high in plant foods and good fats have been proven to be the ultimate combination for prolonging life. Monounsaturated fats, like you find in some nuts and in olive oil, is the main source of fat in the Mediterranean and so much research over the years has shown that this type of fat lowers heart disease, depression, risk of cancer, cognitive decline, inflammatory diseases, and so much more besides – all of which are leading causes of high mortality rates in developed nations.

The Lyon Diet Heart Study was carried out between 1988 and 1992 and focused on people who had suffered heart attacks. They were counseled to either follow a Mediterranean diet or the standard post-heart attack diet, both of which reduce saturated fat. After 4 years, those on the Mediterranean diet experienced up to 70% less heart disease than those on the standard diet – that is three times the risk reduction of those on cholesterol-lowering drugs. They also showed a 45% reduction in risk of death from all causes.

8. It Can Help You to Relax and Lower Stress Levels

The Mediterranean diet encourages followers to commune more with nature, to enjoy meals in the company of others and to sleep better at night. These are all fantastic ways to lower stress and less stress means less inflammation in the body. In general, Mediterranean natives spend more time outdoors and they spend more time with their friends and families, eating good meals and they also make time to enjoy themselves in the garden, dancing, laughing and practicing their hobbies.

We all know that chronic stress is, quite literally, a killer. Your quality of life goes down, your health goes down and your weight goes up and with it comes an increase in the risk of chronic disease. Those who follow the Mediterranean diet enjoy a slower pace, making time to enjoy their meals and to get regular physical activity. Red wine is another part of the diet that is good for the health when consumed in moderation. It has been shown to help fight obesity, among many other things and, added in, the Mediterranean diet is a smart choice for health.

Chapter 3: Myths and Facts Surrounding the Mediterranean Diet

As you saw in the last chapter, the Mediterranean diet has a large number of benefits but it also attracts a lot of misconception on how best to take advantage of this lifestyle for better health and longer, happier life. These are the main myths and facts about the Mediterranean diet:

1. **Myth - It's an expensive diet**

Fact – if you are making your meals from legumes or lentils as the main protein source, and you are sticking to eating mostly whole grain and plant foods, the Mediterranean diet is far less expensive than a pre-packaged processed western diet.

2. **Myth – If one glass of red wine is heart healthy, then surely three glasses is three times healthier**

Fact – nice thinking but only in moderation will you see the benefits of red wine. By moderation, I mean one glass for women and two for men each day, small glasses at that. In moderation, red wine provides some unique heart health benefits but too much and the opposite will be true. More than two glasses of red wine per day can have negative effects on the health of your heart

3. **Myth – Surely the Mediterranean way is lots of bread and large bowls of pasta?**

Fact – Typical Mediterranean do not consume vast amounts of pasta the way Americans do for example. Usually, the pasta will be a small side dish and is no more than ½ to 1 cup in serving size. The rest of the meal consists of vegetables, salad, fish or organic meat and maybe one slice of bread. And that bread will be served with olive oil for dipping, not slathered with butter

4. Myth – If I follow the traditional Mediterranean diet then I will lose weight

Fact – Yes, of course, you will but you have to consider that the traditional Mediterranean dweller, especially those on the Greek islands, don't just eat a good diet. They also spend hours walking up and down hills, often steep ones, to tend their herds and their gardens. They live off of what they produce themselves and physical activity plays a huge part in the success of the diet.

5. Myth – This diet is all about the food

Fact – while the type of food plays a big role, you have to consider the way Mediterranean people actually live their lives. When they eat, they are not eating alone. They don't eat in front of the television or rush their food. Instead, they make meals a relaxed affair, taking time over their food and this is often just as important, if not more, than what you eat.

6. Myth – All vegetable oils are identical and they are all as good for you

Fact – If only it were that simple. There are two different types of unsaturated vegetable oils. First, there are the cold-pressed olive oils and peanut oils that are high in monounsaturated fat, oils that have long been used in the Mediterranean. These are not made with the use of heat or chemicals to extract the oils and, as such, are healthier.

Second, we have the modern oils, the processed oils like sunflower, corn, soybean, canola, cottonseed and vegetable oils. These are manufactured, mainly using genetically modified crops, though the use of toxic solvents and high heat to get the oil out of the seed. This kind of processing can actually damage the nutritional value of the oil and it can turn otherwise healthy fatty acids into trans fats, the most dangerous fats of all. Also, they have a very high content of omega-6 fatty acid and that knocks the balance of omega 3 to omega 6 off kilter, and it is this balance that is crucial to health.

Chapter 4: Ingredients of The Mediterranean Diet

The Mediterranean diet is, as you now know, made up of whole, natural foods. Here are those foods, including their benefits:

Fruits and Vegetables

It is recommended that we eat five portions of vegetables and fruits every day and much of this guidance comes from research into the Mediterranean diet and comes from the WHO. Many governments around the world actually recommend between 7 and 10 portions per day.

Eating a wide range of fresh fruits and vegetables is a vital part of the Mediterranean diet, but tinned, frozen and dried fruits and vegetables also play a part as well. All fruits and vegetables are high in fiber, vitamins, particularly C and antioxidants and have been proven to help reduce the risk of bowel disease, cancer and heart disease.

Cereals

These should be whole grain as far as possible, like wholegrain or whole meal bread, brown pasta or brown rice. Examples of the whole grains you can eat are barley, wheat, rice, corn and millet and these can be found in breakfast cereals, bread, pasta, crackers, and couscous. They provide us with a good dose of complex carbohydrates, fiber, vitamins, protein, and minerals and can also help to fight bowel disease, cancer and can help to lower cholesterol levels, reducing the risk of cardiovascular disease.

Fish

You can eat a range of different fish on the Mediterranean diet, each having their own benefits. For example, white fish is a good source of low-fat protein and includes cod, hake, halibut, plaice, and haddock. Shellfish, like crab, prawns, mussels and lobster contain good levels of protein and trace minerals while oily fish contain high levels of vitamins A and D as well as omega-3 essential fatty acids. It is these acids that can help to lower the risks of heart disease, dementia and some forms of cancer, as well as being helpful in treating depression and in brain development.

Note – Pregnant and nursing women, as well as those who are trying to get pregnant, should be careful about how much shark, tuna and swordfish they eat as these can contain a certain amount of toxic heavy metals.

Legumes

Legumes are vegetables that grow inside pods, like chickpeas, lentils, beans, peas and peanuts. They are an important part of the Mediterranean diet and are useful as bases for stews, soups, hummus and they can easily be eaten on their own. They provide an important source of fiber, carbohydrate, protein and vitamins and are associated with a lower risk of heart disease.

Fats and Oils

When you cook Mediterranean meals, you use monounsaturated fats in place of saturated animal fats. Olive oil is the best and the most traditional oil but you can also use rapeseed oil if you can get it. You will also find these healthy monounsaturated fats in avocado, seeds, nuts, and olives. You can roast your vegetables in a small amount of olive oil and you can use it as a dressing for your salads. Mediterranean people also dip bread in it rather than using butter. Overall, although the levels of fat in the Mediterranean and western diets may be similar, the Mediterranean diet contains much higher levels of monounsaturated fat. However, it should be noted that, no matter what type of fat it is, consuming too much of it may lead to obesity.

Nuts and Seeds

Almonds, walnuts, chestnuts, Brazil nuts, and cashews are all high in the healthy unsaturated fats, as are pumpkin, sesame, sunflower and poppy seeds. They also all contain high livers of vitamins, minerals, protein and fiber. Do avoid salted nuts as these can lead to raised blood pressure and, as with all foods high in fat, too many can lead to obesity.

White Meat

Lean poultry, such as turkey and chicken, are high in minerals, vitamins, and protein so when you cook these meats, remove the skin and trim off any visible fat. White meat that is served in processed foods, such as pies or burger, tends to be higher in animal fat and, as such, should be avoided as an unhealthy choice.

Foods to Eat Occasionally

Some foods can be eaten freely while others, like the ones I list below, should only be eaten occasionally and in small quantities

Wine

Red wine is especially healthy, in moderation. This is often a traditional part of the Mediterranean diet and is good for you because it contains anti-inflammatory chemicals and antioxidants that help to protect the heart. However, it is not good to drink more than one or two small glasses per day, with your meals, as too much will have the opposite effect. Also, wine is full of calories and can cause you to put weight on if you drink too much. Pregnant and nursing women should avoid alcohol altogether.

Dairy Produce

Consumed in small quantities, yogurt, milk, butter, cheese and cream are acceptable on the Mediterranean diet. They contain decent levels of calcium, vitamin A, vitamin B12, and protein. However, some, like butter and cream, are high in saturated fat and should be consumed rarely. Choose cheeses that are low in fat, like feta, mozzarella or cottage cheese over cheddar and cream cheese and choose skimmed or semi-skimmed milk over full fat or cream is better for you.

Red Meat

Red meats like lamb, pork and beef are eaten sparingly on the Mediterranean diet. Although it contains high levels of vitamins, protein, and minerals, it is also much higher in saturated fat than fish and poultry. And, when you find red meat in processed foods, as well as being higher in fat it tends to have a much lower nutritional value. While red meat can be a part of a healthy diet, it is better to keep it as an occasional treat rather than an everyday inclusion in your diet. Think about having it as a roast dinner on Sunday or using it in stews with plenty of vegetables.

Potatoes

Depending on how you cook them, potatoes could be a healthy part of the Mediterranean diet. However, although they contain fiber, potassium, vitamin B and vitamin C, they are also very high in starch. Starch is quickly converted into blood glucose and this raises the risk of type 2 diabetes. Because potatoes don't have the same health benefits of most other vegetables they tend to be kept on a separate list. Boil, bake or mash with butter rather than frying or roasting.

Sweets and Desserts

Sweets foods like sweets, biscuits and cakes are not really a big part of the Mediterranean diet and should only be consumed in small quantities. As well as being high in sugar, they are often much higher in saturated fat. They can have a small amount of nutritional value, for example, a dessert that is milk-based has calcium in it and many desserts do contain fruit but, bearing in mind the level of sugar and other unpleasant ingredients, try to keep them to the absolute minimum.

Portion Guide

This is a basic guide to servings or portion sizes in the Mediterranean diet:

Vegetables: one cup of leafy vegetables (raw) or half a cup of other types of vegetables.

Potatoes: ½ cup.

Legumes: one cup of dry beans, cooked

Nuts: 1/8 cup. Eaten as snacks or sprinkled on your food for a bit of extra taste

Fruit: one apple, one orange, one banana, 1/3 cup grapes, 1 cup watermelon or other melon.

Meat: 2 oz. of lean meat or fish, cooked

Grains: half a cup of cooked pasta or rice; one slice of wholegrain or whole meal bread.

Dairy: one cup of yogurt or milk, ¼ cup of cheese.

Eggs: one whole egg.

Wine: 4-¼ oz. glass of red wine, average strength.

Chapter 5: The Mediterranean Diet Cookbook

So, now you know all about the Mediterranean diet, of what foods you can eat, it's time to take a look at a small selection of recipes to give you an idea of what you can eat on a daily basis.

Breakfast

Mediterranean Couscous

Ingredients

- 3 cups of low-fat milk (maximum 1%)

- 1 cinnamon stick, 2 inches' long

- 1 cup of whole-wheat couscous, uncooked

- ½ cup dried chopped apricots

- ¼ cup dried currants

- 6 tsp dark brown sugar

- ¼ tsp salt

- 4 tsp melted butter

Instructions

- Put the milk and the cinnamon stick into a pan over a medium-high heat and heat up for 3 minutes, or until you see small bubbles around the edge of the pot – do not allow to boil

- Remove the milk from the heat and stir the couscous in

- Add the currants, apricots, salt and 4 tsp brown sugar. Stir well and cover the pan; leave it to stand for 15 minutes

- Remove the cinnamon stick

- Divide the mixture between 4 bowls; drizzle 1 tsp melted butter over the top and sprinkle ½ tsp of brown sugar on before serving immediately

Potato and Chickpea Hash

Ingredients

- 4 cups frozen hash brown potatoes, shredded

- 2 cups baby spinach, finely chopped

- ½ cup onion, finely chopped

- 1 tbsp. fresh ginger, minced

- 1 tbsp. curry powder

- ½ tsp salt

- ¼ cup olive oil, extra-virgin is best

- 1 can chickpeas (15 oz.), drained and rinsed

- 1 cup zucchini, chopped

- 4 whole eggs

Instructions

- Put the shredded potato into a large bowl with the onion, spinach, curry powder, and ginger. Mix together well

- Heat the oil in a large pan and add the potato mixture to it

- Flatten into a layer over the base of the pan and cook until it is crispy golden brown on one side – do not stir.

- Reduce the heat down and fold the zucchini and chickpeas in, breaking up the chunks of potato until everything is combined

- Press the mixture back into a layer and cut 4 dips into it. Break an egg into a cup and pour it into a well; repeat for the other 3.

- Cook until the eggs have set – 4 or 5 minutes for soft yolks, longer for harder ones

Avocado Toast

Ingredients

- 2 small avocados, ripe, peeled and stone removed

- 1/3 cup crumbled soft feta cheese

- 2 tbsp. fresh mint, chopped, plus a little extra for garnish

- A squeeze of fresh lemon for taste

- 4 large slices or rye or whole grain bread

Instructions

- Put the avocado into a bowl and mash using a fork

- Add the mint and lemon juice and mash until combined

- Season with salt and pepper

- Toast the bread and spread ¼ of the avocado on each slice

- Top off with feta and garnish with mint

Pancakes

Ingredients

- 1 cup of old-fashioned oat

- ½ cup of flour, all-purpose

- 2 tbsp. flax seed

- 1 tsp baking soda

- ¼ tsp salt

- 2 cups of plain or vanilla Greek yogurt

- 2 large eggs

- 2 tbsp. organic honey or agave syrup

- Fresh fruit, syrup or other toppings to suit

Instructions

- Combine the oats, flour, salt, baking soda and flax seed together in your blender, pulsing for about 30 seconds

- Add in the eggs, oil, honey and yogurt and blend together until smooth

- Leave to stand for about 20 minutes to thicken up

- Heat up a large pan and brush it with oil

- Ladle ¼ cup of the batter into the skillet and cook until the bottom of the pancake is golden brown; bubbles should be forming on the top of the pancake

- Turn the pancake over and cook for another 2 minutes

- Repeat with the rest of the batter, keeping the pancakes warm in the oven until you have finished

- Serve hot with your favorite toppings

Mediterranean Frittata

Ingredients

- 1 cup of onion, chopped

- 2 cloves minced garlic

- 2 tbsp. olive oil

- 8 eggs

- ¼ cup of light cream, milk or half-and-half

- ½ cup feta cheese, crumbled

- ½ cup of roasted sweet red pepper

- ½ cup of ripe olives, pitted and halved– optional

- ¼ cup fresh basil, slivered

- 1/8 tsp ground black pepper

- ½ cup coarsely crushed onion and garlic croutons

- 2 tbsp. parmesan cheese, finely shredded

- Fresh basil leaves for garnish – optional

Instructions

- Preheat your broiler and heat 2 tbsp. oil in a broiler-proof pan

- Cook the garlic and onion until the onion has just started to turn tender

- Beat the eggs together with the milk and stir the olives, red pepper, feta cheese, black pepper and slivered basil in

- Pour over the onion and garlic in the pan and cook over a medium heat.as it begins to set, loosen the edges off with a spatula, lifting them so the uncooked egg flows underneath

- Continue to do this until all of the mixture has set with a moist surface – do not overcook

- Mix the croutons, the rest of the oil and the parmesan cheese together in a bowl and sprinkle over the frittata mixture

- Broil in the pan, keeping it about 4 or 5 inches from the heat, for 1 or 2 minutes. The top should be set and the crumb mixture golden

- Cut into wedges and serve with a garnish of fresh basil

Lunch

Greek Salad

Ingredients

- 3 large chopped tomatoes

- 2 peeled and chopped cucumbers

- 1 small chopped red onion

- ¼ cup olive oil

- 4 tsp lemon juice

- 1 ½ tsp dried oregano

- Salt and pepper

- 1 cup of feta cheese, crumbled

- 6 large black pitted and sliced olives

Instructions

- Combine the cucumber, tomato, and onion together in a bowl

- Sprinkle the olive oil and lemon juice over the top and season with salt, pepper, and oregano

- Sprinkle the crumbled feta cheese and olives over the salad before serving

Mediterranean Quinoa Salad

Ingredients

- 2 cups water

- 1 smashed garlic clove

- 2 chicken bouillon cubes

- 1 cup quinoa, uncooked

- 2 large chicken breasts, cooked and chopped into small pieces

- 1 large chopped red onion

- 1 large diced green bell pepper

- ½ cup Kalamata olives, chopped

- ½ cup feta cheese, crumbled

- ¼ cup fresh chopped parsley

- ¼ cup fresh chopped chives

- ½ tsp salt

- 2/3 cup of fresh squeezed lemon juice

- 1 tbsp. balsamic vinegar

- ¼ cup olive oil

Instructions

- Put the water, garlic, and bouillon cubes into a pan and bring up to the boil

- Stir the quinoa in, turn the heat down and cover. Simmer for about 15 or 20 minutes, until the quinoa, is tender and all the water has been absorbed

- Remove the smashed garlic clove and transfer the quinoa to a bowl

- Stir the chicken, olives, bell pepper, parsley, feta cheese, chives and salt into the quinoa

- Drizzle the lemon juice, vinegar and olive over the top and stir in thoroughly

- Serve immediately or refrigerate

Creamy White Bean Soup

Ingredients

- 1 tbsp. vegetable oil

- 1 chopped onion

- 1 chopped celery stalk

- 1 clove minced garlic

- 2 cans white kidney beans (16 oz. cans), drained and rinsed

- 1 can chicken broth (14 oz.)

- ¼ tsp black pepper

- 1/8 tsp dried thyme

- 1 bunch fresh rinsed spinach, sliced thinly

- 2 cups water

- 1 tbsp. lemon juice

Instructions

- Heat the oil and cook the celery and onion for about 5 to 8 minutes, or until just soft

- Add the garlic and cook for another 30 seconds, stirring continuously

- Add the beans, pepper, broth, thyme and water, stir well and bring up to the boil

- Turn the heat down and simmer for about 15 minutes

- Using a slotted spoon, take out 2 cups of the beans mixture and set to one side

- Blend the rest of the soup in batches on low speed until it is smooth

- Pour the blended soup into the pan and add back the set aside beans

- Bring up to a boil, stirring occasionally

- Stir the spinach in and cook until the spinach is wilted, about a minute

- Stir the lemon juice in, remove from the heat and serve garnished with grated parmesan cheese

Pasta Fagioli Soup

Ingredients

- 1 can diced tomatoes (29 oz.)

- 2 cans Northern beans (14 oz. each), left undrained

- 1 can chopped and drained spinach (14 oz.)

- 2 cans chicken broth (14 ½ oz. each)

- 1 can tomato sauce (8 oz.)

- 3 cups water

- 1 tbsp. garlic, minced

- 8 slices of crispy bacon, crumbled

- 1 tbsp. dried parsley

- 1 tsp garlic powder

- ½ tsp black pepper

- ½ tsp dried basil

- 1 ½ cups seashell pasta

Instructions

- Put all the ingredients except the pasta into a large pan and stir to combine

- Bring up to a boil and cover the pan, leaving to simmer for 40 minutes

- Add the pasta, cook for about 10 minutes, or until the pasta is tender

- Serve with grated cheese sprinkled over the top

Barley Salad

Ingredients

- 1 cup barley

- 1 sun-dried tomatoes

- 2 ½ cups water

- 2 garlic cloves

- 4 tbsp. olive oil

- 1 tbsp. balsamic vinegar

- ½ cup cilantro finely chopped

- 2/3 cup black olives, chopped

Instructions

- Add the barley and water to a pan and bring to the boil on a high heat

- Reduce the heat, cover the pan and simmer for about 30 minutes, until the barley is firm in the middle but tender

- Drain the barley and set it aside to cool down to room temperature

- Put the tomato, 2 tbsp. oil, the garlic and the balsamic vinegar into your blender and puree until smooth

- Pour it over the barley and fold the olives, cilantro and the rest of the olive oil in

- Cover and refrigerate; serve cold

Dinner

Mediterranean Stew, Slow-Cooker Style

Ingredients

- 1 whole butternut squash, peeled, deseed and cut into cubes

- 2 cups of eggplant, peel on, cubed

- 1 cups zucchini, cubed

- 10 oz. frozen and thawed okra

- 1 8 oz. can tomato sauce

- 1 cup onion, chopped

- 1 ripe chopped tomato

- 1 thin sliced carrot

- ½ cup vegetable broth

- 1/3 cup raisins

- 1 chopped garlic clove

- ½ tsp turmeric powder

- ½ tsp ground cumin

- ¼ tsp red pepper, crushed

- ¼ tsp paprika

Instructions

- Put the squash, eggplant, okra, zucchini, onion, tomato sauce, carrot, tomato, broth, garlic and raisins into the slow cooker

- Season with the spices

- Cook on low for about 8 or 10 hours or until the vegetables are tender

Mediterranean Flounder

Ingredients

- 5 Roma tomatoes

- 2 tbsp. olive oil, extra-virgin is best

- ½ chopped Spanish onion

- A pinch of Italian seasoning

- 24 pitted and chopped Kalamata olives

- ¼ cup white wine

- ¼ cup capers

- 1 tsp fresh squeezed lemon juice

- 12 fresh basil leaves, chopped

- 3 tbsp. parmesan cheese, freshly grated

- 1 lb. fresh flounder fillets

Instructions

- Preheat your oven to 425° F

- Boil a pan of water and plunge in the tomatoes. Immediately put them into a bowl of iced water and then remove the skins

- Chop the de-skinned tomatoes and set to one side

- Heat the oil and sauté the onion for about 5 minutes, or until tender

- Stir the garlic, tomatoes and Italian seasoning in and cook for 5 to 7 minutes, or until the tomatoes are tender

- Mix the wine, olives, capers, lemon juice and half of the basil in, turn the heat down and blend the grated cheese in. Cook for about 15 minutes or until you have a thick sauce

- Put the flounder fillets into a shallow dish and pour the sauce over the top

- Top off with the rest of the basil and bake for about 12 minutes or until the fish flakes easily with a fork

Shrimp Penne

Ingredients

- 16 oz. penne pasta

- ¼ cup red onion, chopped

- 2 tbsp. olive oil

- 1 tbsp. garlic, chopped

- ¼ cup white wine

- 29 oz. canned diced tomatoes

- 1 lb. peeled and deveined shrimp

- 1 cup of parmesan cheese, grated

Instructions

- Salt a pan of water and bring it to the boil

- Add the pasta and cook until it is al dente, about 8 or 10 minutes and then drain it

- Heat the oil and cook the garlic and onion until the onion is tender

- Mix the tomatoes and wine in and cook for about 10 minutes, stirring occasionally

- Mix the shrimp in and cook until opaque, about 5 minutes

- Toss the mixture with the drained pasta and top off with the grated cheese

Greek Chicken Pasta

Ingredients

- 16 oz. linguine pasta

- ½ cup red onion, chopped

- 1 tbsp. olive oil

- 2 crushed garlic cloves

- 1 lb. chicken breast meat, skinless and boneless, chopped into small pieces

- 14 oz. marinated canned artichoke hearts, drained and cut into pieces

- 1 large chopped tomato

- ½ cup feta cheese, crumbled

- 3 tbsp. fresh chopped parsley

- 2 tbsp. freshly squeezed lemon juice

- 2 tsp dried oregano

- Salt and pepper

- 2 wedges of lemon

Instructions

- Salt a pot of water and bring it to the boil

- Cook the pasta until firm but tender, about 8 or 10 minutes, and then drain

- Heat the olive oil and sauté the garlic and onion until fragrant, about 2 minutes

- Stir the chicken in and cook until it is not pink in the middle anymore and the juices are clear, about 5 or 6 minutes

- Turn the heat down and add the artichokes, feta, tomato, lemon juice, parsley, oregano and pasta

- Cook, stirring until it is heated right through, for about 2 or 3 minutes

- Remove the pan from the heat, season and serve garnished with the lemon wedges

Red Pepper and Rosemary Chicken, Slow Cooker Style

Ingredients

- 1 small, thin sliced onion

- 1 red bell pepper, seeded and sliced thinly

- 2 minced garlic cloves

- 2 tsp dried rosemary

- ½ tsp dried oregano

- 8 chicken breast halves, skinless and boneless

- 8 oz. Italian turkey sausage meat

- ¼ tsp coarse black pepper

- 1 ½ tbsp. cornstarch

- ¼ cup dry vermouth

- ¼ cup fresh chopped parsley

- 2 tbsp. cold water

- Salt

Instructions

- Put the onion, garlic, pepper, oregano, and rosemary into a 5 or 6-quart slow cooker and combine together

- Crumble the sausage meat over the top

- Rinse and dry the chicken and place in a single layer over the top

- Sprinkle pepper over the top, pour the vermouth in and put the lid on

- Cook on low for about 5 to 7 hours or until the chicken is tender and cooked through

- Transfer the chicken out of the slow cooker and keep warm

- Mix the cornstarch and water together and stir it into the liquid in the slow cooker

- Turn the heat to high, cover and cook for about 10 minutes, until the sauce has thickened. Stir occasionally to stop it sticking

- Season with salt and serve it over the chicken sprinkled with parsley

Dessert

Orange and Olive Oil Cake

Ingredients

- 2 eggs

- ¾ cup sugar

- 1/3 cup olive oil

- Juice from one orange

- ¾ cups all-purpose flour

- 1 tsp baking powder

- ½ cup whole-wheat pastry flour

- ½ tsp baking soda

- ½ tsp salt

Instructions

- Preheat your oven to 350° F

- Grease and flour a 9-inch cake pan

- Mix the eggs and sugar in a food processor until blended and add the oil, mixing until fully incorporated

- Add the orange juice and mix some more

- In a separate bowl mix the flours, baking soda, baking powder and salt together, whisking to break any lumps up

- Add half of the mixture to the wet mixture and mix on a low speed until combined. Add the rest of the mixture and combine

- Pour the cake batter into the pan and bake for about 25 or 30 minutes, until a toothpick comes out clean

- Leave to cool for at least 15 minutes before serving

Greek Yogurt with Honey, Walnuts, and Figs

Ingredients

- 1 cup of Greek yogurt

- 2 tbsp. toasted chopped walnuts

- 4 fresh figs, cut into quarters

- 2 tbsp. honey

Instructions

- Divide the yogurt between two dishes

- Top off with figs, walnuts and drizzle the honey over the top

Mango-Watermelon Mint Slushy

Ingredients

- 1 cup frozen mango

- 2 cups seedless watermelon, chopped

- ¼ loose packed cup fresh mint leaves, plus extra for garnish

- ¼ tsp salt

- 1 tbsp. sugar

Instructions

- Place all the ingredients into your blender and puree until a smooth consistency

- Serve garnished with fresh mint leaves

Conclusion

I would like to thank you for taking the time to read my book and I hope it has been helpful to you. The Mediterranean diet has been proven time and time again to be one of the healthiest in the world, simply because it is made up of whole foods and good fats, as opposed to the normal western diet, full of processed foods, sugar, salt, trans fats and every other nasty thing you could possibly put into your body.

The Mediterranean diet is not a diet – it is a way of life, one that you will never regret taking up. Even without the inevitable weight loss that will come with the diet, you will feel healthier and you will have so much energy you won't know what to do with it all.

If you have chosen to take on the Mediterranean diet, the next step is to clear your house out of unhealthy foods, clear your mind of unhealthy thoughts and head off to the store with a shopping list. You won't regret the decision and if, like many other people, you are one of those that have tried diet after diet, the Mediterranean diet will make you feel like you have come home after a long absence.

Once again, thank you for reading my book and if you can spare the time, please consider leaving a review for me at Amazon.com

Preview Of "Essential Oils & Aromatherapy - The Ultimate Guide to Improve Health, Reduce Pain and Lose Weight"

Also known as Essential Oil therapy, aromatherapy is the practice of using natural oils extracted from various parts of plants to improve physical and psychological wellbeing. Simply put, aromatherapy seeks to unify your physical, psychological, and spiritual processes to enhance your body's healing process.

The word "aroma" implies the application of natural oils though inhalation to trigger various sensations in the body. While inhalation is an ideal way to use these oils, massaging them onto your body, adding them to your bath water and using them orally (for some varieties of oils) are also acceptable ways of using the oils and deriving their benefits. Due to the effectiveness of natural oils, aromatherapy is an alternative treatment for stress, pain, chronic infections, and weight loss.

Oils used in aromatherapy are widely referred to as essential oils; essential oils come from the leaves, roots, barks, stems, seeds, flowers, and other parts of plants. Specific natural oils have distinct active ingredients that make them useful for a particular purpose. For instance, some oils are effective for physical treatment of problems like acne, swelling, and common fungal infections. Other essential oils such as orange blossom oil are very effective at emotional healing since they relax a troubled mind.

Essential oils are what make the concept of aromatherapy work. As we shall see later, these oils have various benefits. Before we look at how to use essential oils in our day-to-day lives, let us look at how aromatherapy actually works.

To check out the rest of "Essential Oils & Aromatherapy" please search on Amazon for:

"Aromatherapy: Essential Oils & Aromatherapy - The Ultimate Guide to Improve Health, Reduce Pain and Lose Weight "

Or go to:

http://amzn.to/2c8aVUp